Managing Kidney Health Through Nutrition:

A Comprehensive Guide to Combatting Chronic Kidney Disease"

Clifford D. Mason

Table of content

Introduction

Welcome to "Managing Kidney Health Through Nutrition: A Comprehensive Guide to Combatting Chronic Kidney Disease." Within the intricate interplay of health and nutrition lies a transformative opportunity to combat the challenges of Chronic Kidney Disease (CKD). This comprehensive guide is a beacon of empowerment, navigating the labyrinth of nutrition to illuminate the path toward optimal kidney health.

CKD, a global health concern, demands a holistic approach, and the pivotal role of nutrition cannot be overstated. It's within these pages that we embark on an enlightening journey, unveiling the profound impact of dietary choices on kidney function. From decoding the complexities of dietary restrictions to crafting personalized meal plans and embracing transformative lifestyle changes, this guide is a roadmap to reclaiming control over health and vitality.

As we unravel the intricate tapestry of nutrition's influence on CKD, this guide stands as a testament to empowerment. Each chapter unveils insights, strategies, and practical wisdom aimed at empowering individuals to forge a resilient alliance with their health. Through knowledge, informed choices, and proactive engagement, this comprehensive guide aims to empower individuals to wield nutrition as a formidable tool in their battle against CKD.

1. Understanding Chronic Kidney Disease (CKD)

Overview of kidney function

Picture your body as an intricate factory bustling with activity. Among its many departments, the kidneys stand tall as the vigilant janitors, diligently sweeping away waste and maintaining the pristine balance vital for the entire system's harmony.

Step into the grand foyer of these marvelous organs, nestled snugly beneath your rib cage, on a mission that rivals the finest detective's scrutiny. Filtering blood at a staggering rate, these two bean-shaped dynamos process about 120 to 150 quarts of blood daily! Astonishing, isn't it? But that's not all; they sift through this crimson river, siphoning off the waste—sayonara, excess water, toxins, and surplus substances that your body bid farewell to.

Ah, but here comes the real marvel—regulation! Not just satisfied with waste management, the kidneys take charge of the body's fluid balance, akin to an impeccable conductor harmonizing a symphony. They ensure the Goldilocks principle is alive and kicking: not too much, not too little, but just the right amount of water and electrolytes to keep the body's rhythm steady.

Metabolism, that perpetual engine of life, gets its tender loving care from these clever organs. The kidneys play puppeteer to your blood pressure, deftly adjusting it through the release of a hormone named renin. And there's more! They dance with red blood cells, stimulating their production by secreting erythropoietin, ensuring your bloodstream remains vibrant and resilient.

But wait, hold your applause; there's a whisper of caution in this waltz of functions. Picture this wonderland thrown into chaos if these silent heroes falter. Kidney malfunctions can plunge the body into disarray, causing a build-up of waste, triggering high blood pressure, and disrupting the delicate fluid balance. That's when the alarms blare and the entire system suffers.

So, my friends, marvel at the sheer brilliance of these unsung champions—your kidneys! Their multitasking prowess, their finesse in maintaining equilibrium, and their resilience are the threads weaving the fabric of your well-being. They aren't just bean-shaped organs; they are the guardians of equilibrium, the custodians of vitality, ensuring the symphony of life plays on uninterrupted.

Pathophysiology of CKD

Imagine a city where infrastructure crumbles, communication falters, and chaos ensues—a striking analogy to the intricate breakdown witnessed in Chronic Kidney

Disease (CKD). This malady, veiled in silent progression, morphs the vibrant landscape of the kidneys into a battleground of dysfunction.

CKD, a sinister saboteur, tiptoes into the kingdom of these resilient organs, launching its assault on their structural integrity. Initially, it's a covert operation—silent and insidious. Imagine tiny soldiers—nephrons, the kidney's fundamental units—under siege. Scar tissue creeps in, reducing their numbers, while inflammation wreaks havoc, impairing their ability to function seamlessly.

The residents—your body's lifeblood—find themselves at the mercy of this turmoil. Waste, normally escorted out like unruly guests, starts lingering, contaminating the purity of the bloodstream. Picture the fluid balance teetering, like a delicate scale now tipped awry—too much or too little, both dire straits for the body's equilibrium.

But that's not all. The hormonal harmony orchestrated by these guardians crumbles. Renin, the blood pressure conductor, often overplays its hand, resulting in the rise of hypertension—a menacing ally to CKD. Meanwhile, the production of erythropoietin dwindles, dimming the vitality of red blood cells, plunging the body into a state of perpetual fatigue.

The domino effect unfurls—a relentless cascade of complications. Bones, robbed of their guardians' mineral-balancing act, weaken, prone to fractures and fractures. Acid-base balance spirals out of control, triggering a pH rollercoaster ride detrimental to the body's stability.

Alas, the consequences aren't confined to the confines of the kidneys alone. CKD, the master of disguise, masquerades as a puppeteer pulling strings across the body. It snags the cardiovascular system, weaving a tapestry of heart disease and stroke, and stealthily tugs at the metabolic strings, fostering diabetes and dyslipidemia.

But fear not! Awareness emerges as the beacon of hope. Early detection, lifestyle tweaks, and medical interventions—these are the glimmers of light that can tame this mighty beast. A symphony of medication, dietary adjustments, and sometimes, the miraculous transplant—the tools to defy CKD's relentless advance.

In this chronicle of affliction, understanding the pathophysiology unravels the mystery behind CKD's relentless progression. It sheds light on the chaos brewing within, empowering us to marshal our forces—medical, dietary, and proactive—to shield the kingdom of our kidneys from the perils of this chronic assailant.

Identifying Signs and Symptoms

In the labyrinth of our bodies, signs and symptoms serve as guiding stars, offering clues to the brewing storms within. When it comes to Chronic Kidney Disease (CKD), these harbingers often tiptoe in, whispering their presence before the tempest gathers.

Picture this: an unrelenting fatigue creeping into your days, as if carrying an invisible weight upon your shoulders. Your body, a marvel of balance, starts betraying signs—swollen ankles and feet, a consequence of the body's struggle to balance fluids. Unquenchable thirst and an incessant need to visit the restroom more frequently—these too are the messengers of CKD.

The subtlety of these symptoms, akin to a soft-spoken prologue, often goes unnoticed, camouflaged amidst the clamor of daily life. But they persist, nudging us to pay heed, to look deeper.

The insidious nature of CKD lends it the guise of a silent assassin. Often, it takes a toll on the body stealthily, masquerading behind seemingly innocuous signs until it reaches more advanced stages. Elevated blood pressure might whisper of the kidneys' silent distress, urging a closer examination.

Ah, but there's more to this tale of warning! The very chemistry of your blood, the orchestra of your body's wellness, might reveal the crescendo of CKD. Elevated levels of creatinine or urea, the waste products normally whisked away by the kidneys, serve as red flags—an SOS from the body's inner sanctum.

As the malaise deepens, symptoms grow bolder, more pronounced. Picture a loss of appetite, a metallic taste lingering in your mouth, muscle cramps tightening their grip—a cacophony of distress signals emitted by a body battling the encroaching shadows of CKD.

Yet, amid this ominous backdrop, there shines a beacon of hope—early detection. Regular health check-ups and vigilance empower us to decipher these cryptic signs, to heed their whispers before they crescendo into a symphony of irreversible damage.

Understanding these telltale signs becomes our shield, our safeguard against the stealthy advances of CKD. It's the roadmap guiding us through the labyrinth, enabling us to intercept, intervene, and safeguard the sanctity of our kidneys—the silent sentinels of our well-being.

2. The Role of Nutrition in Kidney Health

Impact of Diet on CKD Progression

Oh, the canvas of health, where each and every bite contributes a stroke to the well-being masterpiece that is being created! When it comes to Chronic Kidney Disease (CKD), the palette of nutrition exerts a deep effect; it is a powerful brush that shapes the evolution of this silent invader and the treatment of it.

Imagine your dietary choices as architects, crafting the foundation upon which CKD treads. Sodium, that ubiquitous mineral, when in excess, plays the role of a saboteur, escalating blood pressure and triggering fluid retention. Picture the kidneys, burdened by this excess, straining under the weight of their duties.

Yet, it's not just sodium—protein, the building block of life, too, holds a pivotal role. In the intricate dance of CKD, excessive protein can transform into a double-edged sword, taxing the kidneys' filtration capacity. The delicate balance between providing nourishment and burdening these overworked guardians requires a masterful choreography.

Phosphorus and potassium, often lurking stealthily in everyday foods, emerge as silent accomplices in CKD's progression. Elevated levels, a consequence of dietary indulgence, spell trouble for the body's mineral harmony. Picture the skeletal system, disrupted by excess phosphorus, weakening its fortitude.

But behold, the hero emerges—nutritional intervention! A symphony of moderation, precision, and strategic selection transforms the dietary landscape. Limiting sodium intake becomes the cornerstone—a guardian angel easing the burden on beleaguered kidneys, curbing the perilous dance of blood pressure.

Ah, but it doesn't stop there! Pruning excessive protein, akin to trimming unruly branches, lightens the filtration load on the kidneys, safeguarding their dwindling functionality. The art of balancing phosphorus and potassium, a tightrope act in the nutritional circus, demands meticulous attention—a feat achievable through prudent food choices and portion control.

Behold the magic of the Mediterranean diet—its heart-healthy bounty of fruits, vegetables, whole grains, and lean proteins emerges as a soothing balm for CKD. Its gentle embrace of moderation, its melody of nutrient-rich, low-phosphorus foods, orchestrates a serenade to the ailing kidneys.

The impact of diet on CKD transcends mere sustenance. It morphs into a formidable tool, a healer guiding the trajectory of this malady. Empowered by knowledge and armed with prudent dietary choices, we embark on a transformative journey—one that nurtures, supports, and shields the delicate dance of the kidneys, steering them away from the perils of CKD's relentless advance.

Renal-Friendly Foods and Their Benefits

The culinary symphony that was produced to calm the tired kidneys is a melodious tapestry that is woven with foods that are favorable to the kidneys. Each note is a blessing in the fight against the looming shadows of Chronic Kidney Disease (CKD).

Behold the almighty hero: the bounty of fruits and vegetables! Picture them as nature's medicine chest, laden with antioxidants, vitamins, and minerals. Their low potassium and phosphorus content make them the revered pillars of renal wellness. Crisp apples, vibrant berries, crunchy bell peppers, and leafy greens emerge as guardians, their vibrant hues concealing a treasure trove of nourishment.

Lean proteins, the valiant knights of this nutritional saga, take center stage. Tender cuts of chicken, fish, and eggs step forth as saviors, their moderate protein content offering sustenance without burdening the faltering kidneys. Picture them as the cornerstone of a renal-friendly feast, their role pivotal in maintaining muscle strength without taxing filtration.

Whole grains, the unsung heroes gracing the table, bring forth their bounty of fiber and nutrients. Their modest phosphorus content and fiber-rich nature offer a double-edged sword of protection—nurturing the body while sparing the kidneys from undue stress. Embrace the wholesome embrace of oats, quinoa, and brown rice, for they fortify the body's fortress against CKD's advances.

Enter the symphony of herbs and spices—a dazzling array of flavors that elevate renal-friendly dishes without compromising on taste. Their magical touch infuses zest into meals while sidestepping the pitfalls of excessive sodium. Marvel at the potency of rosemary, basil, and turmeric, their culinary prowess transcending mere seasoning to bestow healing benefits.

Behold the triumphant return of calcium! Despite the cautionary whispers surrounding phosphorus, the judicious inclusion of calcium-rich foods holds sway. Picture low-fat dairy products like yogurt and cheese, their calcium content offsetting the harmful effects of excess phosphorus, safeguarding the body's skeletal integrity.

But amidst this feast of abundance, hydration emerges as the unsung champion—a simple elixir with profound effects. Water, the elixir of life, dances gracefully, flushing away toxins and maintaining the body's fluid balance. Its prowess in supporting kidney function cannot be overstated, making it a cornerstone of renal-friendly diets.

Renal-friendly foods emerge not merely as sustenance but as healers, nurturers, and guardians. Their gentle embrace, rich in nutrients yet mindful of the kidney's vulnerabilities, stands as a testament to the power of food in steering the body away from the turbulent waters of CKD. Armed with knowledge and guided by these nourishing allies, we embark on a transformative journey—a journey that celebrates the harmony between food and renal wellness.

Effect of Lifestyle Choices on Kidney Function

Every decision we make and every routine we engage in creates a narrative that reverberates throughout the hallowed chambers of our kidneys. Oh, the exquisite tapestry that is our way of life. When it comes to shielding these strong organs from the assault of diseases like Chronic Kidney Disease (CKD), lifestyle appears as the maestro orchestrating the symphony of their well-being.

The pulse that invigorates the body and infuses energy into every nook of our being is the rhythm of physical activity. Behold with me the rhythm of physical activity. Exercise on a consistent basis is not only a reliable indicator of cardiovascular health, but it also serves as a strong protective mechanism for renal function. In addition to flushing out impurities and maintaining the kidneys' vitality, its regular cadence and dance with circulation ensure that the kidneys continue to fulfill their job as watchful guards of our internal homeostasis.

Oh, but as we make our way through the maze of nutrition, the narrative becomes more complicated. Every choice we make, whether it be with the meals we consume or the fluids we consume, has repercussions within the delicate constraints of our renal landscape. Excessive salt, the omnipresent visitor in our meals, heightens blood pressure and alters fluid balance, tilting the scales against kidney health. Picture the wicked duo—sugary drinks and processed foods—nurturing inflammation, paving the path for CKD's stealthy development.

Yet, the story isn't one of deprivation, but of empowerment. Behold the transformational power of a balanced diet—rich in fruits, vegetables, lean meats, and whole grains. Its nourishing embrace fortifies the body, placing onto the kidneys a barrier against the ravages of sickness. Hydration emerges as the elixir of life—a simple but effective ally, washing away pollutants and sustaining the delicate balance inside.

Behold, too, the shadowy figures lurking in the haze of lifestyle choices—cigarette smoke and excess alcohol. Their assault on kidney function is as stealthy as it is severe. Tobacco's malevolent dance with blood vessels tightens the noose around the kidneys, while alcohol, a deceptive elixir, disrupts their delicate filtration process, spelling trouble for their resilience.

But lo and behold, the guiding light—stress management! The maestro of our mental well-being, stress, when left unchecked, orchestrates a symphony of hormonal havoc. Its relentless grip elevates blood pressure, triggers inflammation, and destabilizes the body's equilibrium—a perilous path that encumbers the kidneys in their noble duties.

Lifestyle emerges not merely as a series of choices but as the conductor guiding the symphony of kidney function. Its harmonious blend of exercise, balanced nutrition, hydration, and stress management becomes the lighthouse, illuminating the path toward renal wellness. Empowered by awareness and armed with proactive choices, we embark on a transformative journey—one that celebrates the harmonious dance between lifestyle and the resilient guardians of our well-being, our kidneys.

3. Nutritional Strategies for Managing CKD

Dietary Modifications in Different Stages of CKD

The evolving landscape of dietary modifications—tailored orchestrations to navigate the ever-shifting tides of Chronic Kidney Disease (CKD). Picture it as a grand tapestry woven with nuances, each stage of CKD demanding a unique culinary symphony to safeguard the delicate dance of the kidneys.

In the early stages, when CKD tiptoes in like a whisper, dietary interventions serve as the heralds of defense. Sodium reduction emerges as the cornerstone, a shield against the impending assault on blood pressure and fluid balance. Imagine the gentle pruning of high-sodium foods, a stride toward stability in the body's equilibrium.

Ah, but as the saga progresses, the plot thickens. Enter the realm of moderate protein intake—a delicate balancing act. The kidneys, already burdened, call for prudence in protein consumption. Precision becomes the mandate—a fine-tuning of protein quantities to support the body's needs while sparing the faltering kidneys undue filtration strain.

As CKD unfurls its malevolent tendrils, phosphorus and potassium emerge as the antagonists in this culinary saga. Their excesses, concealed within everyday foods, pose a threat to the body's mineral harmony. Picture the meticulous choreography—limiting high-phosphorus foods like dairy and nuts, moderating potassium-rich fare like bananas and potatoes—each step aimed at preserving the dwindling balance.

But behold, the crescendo of advanced CKD—the stage where dietary modifications assume an even more pivotal role. Here, the orchestra shifts its tempo. Potassium and phosphorus restriction becomes more stringent, a necessary sacrifice to preserve the fragile equilibrium within the body. Imagine the meticulous scrutiny of every morsel, the careful curation of a meal plan designed to shield the besieged kidneys.

Yet, amid this daunting landscape, a guiding light emerges—the golden rule of fluid management. As CKD advances, the body's ability to regulate fluids wanes. The symphony of hydration, once a simple melody, transforms into a delicate ballet—each sip measured, each drop accounting for the body's intricate balance.

Dietary modifications assume the role of healers, guardians, and custodians of renal wellness. They adapt, evolve, and transform with each stage of CKD, orchestrating a symphony that nurtures, sustains, and shields the delicate dance of the kidneys.

Armed with knowledge and guided by these culinary interventions, we embark on a transformative journey—one that celebrates the harmony between dietary modifications and the resilient guardians of our well-being, our kidneys.

Renal Diet Guidelines and Restrictions

The intricate dance of renal diet guidelines and restrictions—a labyrinthine tapestry woven with precision to safeguard the delicate equilibrium within the kingdom of the kidneys. Picture it as a symphony—a harmonious blend of guidelines and limitations meticulously crafted to nurture renal wellness amidst the tempest of Chronic Kidney Disease (CKD).

Enter the cornerstone of this dietary saga: sodium reduction. Its omnipresence in the modern diet serves as a formidable adversary, threatening the balance of blood pressure and fluid retention. Renal guidelines advocate for a trim in sodium intake, an artful pruning of high-sodium culprits—processed foods, canned goods, and salty indulgences—ushering in stability in the body's delicate equilibrium.

Ah, but the plot thickens with the mandate of protein moderation—a delicate tightrope walk. In the realm of CKD, excessive protein burdens the faltering kidneys, straining their filtration capacity. Renal guidelines steer toward moderation, a measured approach that maintains the body's muscle strength without exacerbating the kidneys' plight.

Behold the silent assailants—phosphorus and potassium—lurking within everyday foods. Their excesses, a looming threat to mineral balance, necessitate vigilant restrictions. Renal guidelines unfurl their wisdom, urging a meticulous curation of meals that minimize high-phosphorus foods like dairy and nuts, while taming potassium-rich indulgences such as bananas and potatoes.

Fluid management emerges as the linchpin—a delicate balancing act. As CKD advances, the body's ability to regulate fluids diminishes. Renal guidelines delineate precise fluid allowances, guiding every sip to maintain the delicate equilibrium without overwhelming the beleaguered kidneys.

Yet, amid these stringent dictates, a glimmer of sustenance emerges—balanced nutrition. Renal guidelines advocate for a tableau rich in fruits, vegetables, lean proteins, and whole grains, fostering nourishment while treading the fine line of restrictions. Embracing the bounty of renal-friendly foods becomes the anthem, nurturing the body's fortitude against CKD's advances.

Renal diet guidelines and restrictions unfurl as the guardians, custodians, and healers of renal wellness. They choreograph a symphony of nourishment and caution, empowering individuals to embrace a culinary narrative that nurtures, sustains, and shields the delicate dance of the kidneys.

Importance of Monitoring Nutrient Levels

The vigilant guardianship bestowed upon our bodies—monitoring nutrient levels emerges as the sentinel, the watchful eye that ensures the delicate balance within the intricate landscape of our health, especially in the realm of Chronic Kidney Disease (CKD).

Picture this monitoring as a compass, guiding us through the labyrinth of CKD's challenges. Nutrient levels, the vital markers adorning this compass, offer a roadmap—a glimpse into the body's inner sanctum. Creatinine and urea levels, akin to loyal sentinels, stand as indicators of the kidneys' filtration prowess, whispering clues about their functionality.

Ah, but delve deeper! Electrolytes—potassium, sodium, phosphorus—they emerge as the guardians of mineral harmony. Monitoring their levels becomes a crucial mandate, a beacon warning of any disturbances that could disrupt the body's delicate equilibrium. Elevated potassium, for instance, might signal kidney distress, while heightened phosphorus levels might herald skeletal threats.

Yet, it's not merely about surveillance; it's about proactive intervention. Regular monitoring allows for early detection of imbalances, enabling timely interventions to stave off CKD's relentless march. It empowers healthcare professionals to tweak dietary plans, adjust medications, or explore interventions before these imbalances snowball into larger complications.

In this saga of vigilant oversight, monitoring nutrient levels transcends mere observation; it becomes a lifeline—a tool that empowers individuals and healthcare providers alike. It fosters a proactive approach, a partnership between awareness and intervention, to safeguard the delicate dance of the kidneys.

Imagine this monitoring as a symphony conductor, orchestrating harmony within the body's biochemical orchestra. Its keen eye ensures that the melodies of nutrient levels remain in perfect cadence, warding off the dissonance that CKD might seek to sow.

4. Designing a Kidney-Friendly Diet Plan

Meal Planning Techniques

The culinary artistry of meal planning—a tapestry woven with precision, creativity, and foresight. In the realm of Chronic Kidney Disease (CKD), meal planning emerges not just as a culinary chore but as a powerful tool—a guiding compass that navigates the delicate dance of nutrition while honoring the restrictions imposed by the condition.

Enter the cornerstone of this culinary symphony—portion control. Imagine it as the architect, meticulously sculpting meals to strike a balance between nourishment and restriction. Portion control becomes the guiding principle, ensuring moderation in protein, phosphorus, potassium, and sodium intake, safeguarding the besieged kidneys.

The blueprint for renal meal planning unfurls with the guiding light of moderation. It's about embracing the bounty of fruits, vegetables, whole grains, and lean proteins while judiciously trimming the excesses lurking within—phosphorus-rich dairy, potassium-laden bananas, and sodium-laden processed foods.

Variety becomes the maestro's baton—a celebration of diverse flavors and textures. The canvas of meal planning paints a panorama that thrives on diversity, ensuring a rich array of nutrients while sidestepping monotony. Picture the vibrant hues of assorted vegetables, the melody of grains, and the dance of proteins gracing the plate in a symphony of culinary delight.

Oh, but the plot thickens with strategic swaps and substitutions! In the culinary theater of CKD, creativity reigns supreme. Low-phosphorus dairy alternatives, potassium-conscious produce choices, and sodium-restricted seasonings step forth as the heroes—innovative tools to craft flavorful, kidney-friendly feasts.

Timing emerges as the choreographer's cue—a delicate synchronization of meals throughout the day. Spreading out nutrient intake becomes the mandate, ensuring a gentle ebb and flow of nourishment without overwhelming the kidneys. Picture it as a ballet—breakfast, lunch, dinner, and snacks orchestrated with precision, honoring the body's rhythms.

And behold, the beacon of preparation! Meal planning flourishes with thoughtful preparation—batch cooking, pre-cutting ingredients, and mindful storage become the pillars. They streamline the culinary process, transforming it into a seamless experience, ensuring adherence to the nutritional roadmap laid out.

Meal planning emerges not just as a chore but as an art—a tapestry woven with foresight, creativity, and precision. It nurtures, sustains, and shields the delicate dance of the kidneys, empowering individuals to embrace a flavorful, nourishing, and renal-friendly culinary narrative.

Tailoring Diet to Individual Needs

The culinary tapestry tailored to the individual—a personalized symphony resonating with the unique nuances of health, preferences, and challenges. In the realm of Chronic Kidney Disease (CKD), the art of tailoring diets to individual needs transcends a mere culinary chore; it becomes a transformative journey that honors the intricacies of each person's health landscape.

Enter the cornerstone of this bespoke culinary narrative—personalization. Each individual, a unique canvas, demands a dietary masterpiece sculpted to their specific needs. Personalization unfolds as the guiding principle—a tailored roadmap that navigates the labyrinth of CKD, accounting for medical history, kidney function, nutritional requirements, and taste preferences.

The first brushstroke in this culinary canvas—medical history and kidney function. A careful examination of renal health, alongside any accompanying conditions, guides the crafting of a nutritional roadmap. It identifies the degree of kidney function, the presence of complications, and sets the stage for a personalized dietary intervention.

Ah, but it's not merely about health parameters; it's about celebrating preferences. Picture this culinary portrait embracing individual tastes, cultural backgrounds, and lifestyle choices. It's about sculpting meals that resonate with familiarity and comfort—a culinary journey that harmonizes the flavors of tradition with the needs of renal health.

Portion control emerges as the palette—meticulously tailored to the individual's needs. For some, it might involve meticulous measurements to balance protein, phosphorus, potassium, and sodium intake. For others, it might encompass visual cues or hand portions, honoring individual habits while adhering to nutritional guidelines.

Flexibility becomes the linchpin—a flexible approach that accommodates changes in health status, preferences, and even seasonal availability of foods. It's a living, breathing canvas that adapts, evolves, and reshapes itself in accordance with the individual's journey through CKD.

Educational support plays a pivotal role—a companion on this journey. Empowering individuals with knowledge about renal health, nutrition, and the impact of dietary choices nurtures a deeper understanding, fostering an active partnership in the process of personalizing their diets.

Tailoring diets to individual needs transcends mere nourishment; it becomes a transformative journey. It honors the uniqueness of each person's health landscape, celebrates preferences, and empowers individuals to embrace a culinary narrative that nurtures, sustains, and shields the delicate dance of their kidneys. s.

Recipes and Meal Ideas for Kidney Health

Let's delve into a culinary journey that celebrates the flavors, nourishment, and kidney-friendly delights! Here's a spectrum of recipes and meal ideas meticulously crafted to nurture renal wellness amidst the tapestry of Chronic Kidney Disease (CKD).

1. Grilled Lemon Herb Chicken:

Marinate chicken breasts in a mixture of lemon juice, olive oil, garlic, and herbs.

Grill until cooked through and serve with a side of roasted vegetables and quinoa for a nutrient-rich meal.

2. Vegetable Stir-Fry with Tofu:

Sauté colorful vegetables—bell peppers, broccoli, carrots, and snap peas—with tofu in a low-sodium sauce.

Serve over brown rice for a balanced and kidney-friendly delight.

3. Salmon with Herbed Yogurt Sauce:

Bake salmon fillets and top them with a refreshing sauce made from Greek yogurt, dill, lemon juice, and garlic.

Pair with a side of steamed asparagus and a quinoa salad for a protein-rich feast.

4. Eggplant Parmesan:

Create a lighter version by baking eggplant slices instead of frying.

Layer with low-sodium marinara sauce and a sprinkle of reduced-fat mozzarella cheese. Bake until golden and bubbly.

5. Bean and Vegetable Chili:

Make a hearty chili using kidney beans, black beans, diced tomatoes, bell peppers, onions, and lean ground turkey or chicken. Season with kidney-friendly herbs and spices like cumin, oregano, and chili powder.

6. Rainbow Fruit Salad:

Combine a variety of kidney-friendly fruits such as berries, apples, grapes, and citrus fruits in a colorful salad. Add a drizzle of honey or a sprinkle of chopped mint for extra flavor.

7. Mediterranean Veggie Wrap:

Fill a whole-grain wrap with hummus, sliced cucumbers, tomatoes, shredded carrots, mixed greens, and a sprinkle of feta cheese.

Roll it up for a delicious, kidney-friendly lunch option.

8. Quinoa and Roasted Vegetable Bowl:

Roast a medley of vegetables like zucchini, bell peppers, cherry tomatoes, and red onions.

Toss with cooked quinoa and a drizzle of balsamic glaze for a flavorful and nutrient-packed bowl.

9. Herbed Chicken and Vegetable Skewers:

Thread marinated chicken chunks, cherry tomatoes, mushrooms, and bell peppers onto skewers.

Grill until cooked and serve with a side of couscous or brown rice.

10. Low-Phosphorus Banana Pancakes:

Make pancakes using a low-phosphorus flour alternative and mashed bananas.

Serve with a dollop of Greek yogurt and fresh berries for a kidney-friendly breakfast.

These recipes and meal ideas celebrate the abundance of flavors while adhering to renal-friendly guidelines. They embrace a balance of nutrients, creativity, and culinary delight, nurturing the delicate dance of the kidneys amidst the journey through CKD.

5. Breakfasts for Kidney Health

Low-Phosphorus Breakfast Dishes

Crafting a low-phosphorus breakfast repertoire celebrates culinary creativity while honoring the restrictions imposed by Chronic Kidney Disease (CKD). Here's a spread of delightful breakfast dishes meticulously tailored to be kind to your kidneys:

1. Oatmeal with Fresh Fruit:

Start your day with a bowl of oatmeal made with water or a low-phosphorus milk alternative.
Top it with kidney-friendly fruits like berries, sliced apples, or pears for a burst of flavor and added nutrition.

2. Egg White Omelette:

Whip up an omelette using egg whites and incorporate kidney-friendly veggies such as spinach, bell peppers, and onions.

Season with herbs and spices for added flavor without the phosphorus.

3. Yogurt Parfait with Nuts and Seeds:

Opt for a low-phosphorus yogurt or Greek yogurt and layer it with chopped nuts and seeds like almonds or chia seeds.
Add a drizzle of honey or a sprinkle of cinnamon for extra sweetness and flavor.

4. Smoothie Bowl:

Blend together a smoothie using low-phosphorus fruits such as berries, peaches, or mangoes, along with a banana or avocado for creaminess.
Pour it into a bowl and top with kidney-friendly toppings like granola, coconut flakes, or pumpkin seeds.

5. Low-Phosphorus Pancakes or Waffles:

Make pancakes or waffles using a low-phosphorus flour alternative and serve them with a topping of fresh fruit or a drizzle of low-phosphorus syrup.

6. Toasted Whole Grain Bread with Avocado:

Toast whole grain bread and top it with mashed avocado for a creamy and nutrient-packed breakfast.
Sprinkle with herbs, salt, and pepper for added flavor.

7. Homemade Low-Phosphorus Granola:

Bake a batch of homemade granola using low-phosphorus ingredients like oats, unsweetened coconut flakes, and nuts/seeds like sunflower or pumpkin seeds.
Enjoy it with a low-phosphorus milk or yogurt for a crunchy and satisfying breakfast.

8. Low-Phosphorus Muffins or Scones:

Bake muffins or scones using a low-phosphorus flour alternative and incorporate kidney-friendly fruits like blueberries or cranberries.

9. Rice Cake or Corn Cake with Nut Butter:

Spread a rice cake or corn cake with a kidney-friendly nut butter like almond or cashew butter for a quick and easy breakfast option.

10. Veggie Breakfast Hash:

Sauté kidney-friendly vegetables such as bell peppers, zucchini, and spinach and serve them with scrambled egg whites or tofu for a hearty breakfast dish.

These low-phosphorus breakfast ideas embrace a variety of flavors, textures, and nutrients, offering a delightful start to your day while being mindful of your kidney health.

Breakfast Bowls and Porridge Varieties

Breakfast bowls and porridges offer a canvas for a myriad of flavors and textures while catering to different dietary needs, including those of individuals managing Chronic Kidney Disease (CKD). Here's a variety of wholesome breakfast bowls and porridge options that are versatile, nutritious, and can be adapted to meet low-phosphorus requirements:

1. Fruit and Nut Porridge:
Prepare a base of low-phosphorus grains like oats or quinoa cooked in water or a low-phosphorus milk alternative.
Top it with kidney-friendly fruits such as berries, sliced apples, or pears, and add a sprinkle of chopped nuts or seeds for crunch and added nutrients.

2. Savory Breakfast Bowl:

Cook a base of low-phosphorus grains like brown rice or barley.

Top it with kidney-friendly vegetables such as sautéed spinach, roasted tomatoes, and caramelized onions. Add a poached egg or tofu for protein.

3. Coconut Chia Seed Pudding:

Mix chia seeds with a low-phosphorus milk alternative and unsweetened coconut flakes. Let it sit in the fridge overnight to thicken. Top it with kidney-friendly fruits like mangoes or kiwi for a refreshing breakfast bowl.

4. Quinoa Breakfast Bowl:

Cook quinoa in water or a low-phosphorus liquid and layer it with kidney-friendly fruits such as sliced bananas, blueberries, and a drizzle of honey or maple syrup.

5. Sorghum Breakfast Porridge:

Use sorghum as a base for a hearty porridge cooked with water or a low-phosphorus liquid.

Top it with roasted nuts, diced apples, and a sprinkle of cinnamon for a comforting breakfast bowl.

6. Tropical Smoothie Bowl:

Blend frozen low-phosphorus fruits like pineapple, mango, and banana with a splash of low-phosphorus liquid.

Pour it into a bowl and top it with kidney-friendly toppings such as shredded coconut, sliced kiwi, and granola for a refreshing breakfast option.

7. Millet Breakfast Bowl:

Cook millet in water or a low-phosphorus liquid and serve it with kidney-friendly toppings like diced peaches, chopped almonds, and a touch of cinnamon or nutmeg.

8. Buckwheat Porridge:
Cook buckwheat groats in water or a low-phosphorus liquid until tender.
Top it with kidney-friendly toppings like berries, sliced figs, and a dollop of Greek yogurt or a non-dairy alternative.

9. Amaranth Breakfast Bowl:
Cook amaranth in water or a low-phosphorus liquid and layer it with kidney-friendly fruits such as raspberries, blackberries, and a sprinkle of sunflower seeds for added crunch.

10. Protein-Packed Breakfast Bowl:
Combine cooked quinoa or lentils with kidney-friendly vegetables, diced tofu or shredded chicken for protein, and top it with a drizzle of low-phosphorus sauce or dressing.

These breakfast bowls and porridges offer a spectrum of flavors, nutrients, and textures, allowing for a creative and nourishing start to the day while catering to kidney-friendly dietary requirements.

Egg-Free Protein Breakfasts

Egg-free protein-rich breakfasts offer a diverse array of options for those seeking alternatives to eggs while ensuring adequate protein intake. Here are some delicious and protein-packed breakfast ideas without eggs:

1. Greek Yogurt Parfait:

Layer low-fat Greek yogurt with mixed berries, chopped nuts, and a sprinkle of granola or seeds for a protein-rich and flavorful breakfast.

2. Chia Seed Pudding:

Mix chia seeds with a low-phosphorus milk alternative and a touch of sweetener. Refrigerate overnight for a creamy pudding loaded with protein and topped with fresh fruit or nuts.

3. Tofu Scramble:

Sauté crumbled tofu with vegetables like spinach, bell peppers, and onions.
Season with herbs and spices for a savory and protein-packed alternative to scrambled eggs.

4. Protein Smoothie Bowl:

Blend together a protein-rich smoothie using a low-phosphorus milk or yogurt, banana, spinach, and a scoop of protein powder.
Pour into a bowl and top it with nuts, seeds, and fresh fruit for added texture and nutrients.

5. Cottage Cheese Breakfast Bowl:

Enjoy cottage cheese with sliced fruits like peaches, pineapple, or berries.
Sprinkle with nuts or seeds for a protein-rich and satisfying breakfast.

6. Hummus Toast:

Spread hummus on whole-grain toast and top it with sliced tomatoes, cucumber, and a drizzle of olive oil.

Sprinkle with seeds or nuts for an added protein boost.

7. Nut Butter Overnight Oats:

Mix rolled oats with a low-phosphorus liquid and a spoonful of nut butter.

Refrigerate overnight and top it with sliced bananas, berries, and a sprinkle of seeds or nuts.

8. Quinoa Breakfast Bowl:

Cook quinoa in water or a low-phosphorus liquid and top it with roasted vegetables, avocado, and a drizzle of tahini or a nut-based sauce for protein.

9. Plant-Based Protein Pancakes:

Prepare pancakes using a combination of protein-rich ingredients like chickpea flour, mashed bananas, or protein powder.

Serve them with a dollop of Greek yogurt or a non-dairy alternative and fresh fruit.

10. Protein-Packed Smoothie:
Blend together a smoothie using a low-phosphorus milk, frozen fruits, spinach or kale, a scoop of protein powder, and a spoonful of nut butter.
Enjoy a nutritious and protein-filled breakfast on-the-go.

These egg-free protein breakfast options offer a delightful variety, catering to different tastes and dietary preferences while ensuring a hearty start to the day.

6. Satisfying Lunch Options

Salads with Kidney-Friendly Dressings

Crafting flavorful salads with kidney-friendly dressings ensures a delightful balance of taste and renal wellness. Here are some delicious salad ideas paired with kidney-friendly dressings:

1. Mixed Greens Salad with Balsamic Vinaigrette:

Toss mixed greens, cherry tomatoes, cucumbers, and sliced bell peppers in a bowl.

Drizzle with a kidney-friendly balsamic vinaigrette made from balsamic vinegar, olive oil, a touch of honey, and herbs like basil or thyme.

2. Mediterranean Chickpea Salad with Lemon-Tahini Dressing:

Combine chickpeas, chopped cucumbers, cherry tomatoes, red onions, and olives in a bowl.

Drizzle with a kidney-friendly lemon-tahini dressing made from tahini, lemon juice, garlic, and a splash of water for consistency.

3. Quinoa and Vegetable Salad with Herb Dressing:

Mix cooked quinoa with diced bell peppers, shredded carrots, chopped parsley, and diced red onions.

Toss with a kidney-friendly herb dressing made from olive oil, lemon juice, fresh herbs like dill or parsley, and a touch of Dijon mustard.

4. Kale and Berry Salad with Yogurt Dressing:

Massage kale leaves with a bit of olive oil, then toss with kidney-friendly berries like strawberries or blueberries.

Top with a kidney-friendly yogurt dressing made from Greek yogurt, honey, a splash of lemon juice, and a pinch of cinnamon.

5. Tomato and Mozzarella Salad with Pesto Dressing:

Arrange sliced tomatoes, fresh mozzarella, and basil leaves on a plate.
Drizzle with a kidney-friendly pesto dressing made from basil, pine nuts, garlic, olive oil, and a sprinkle of Parmesan cheese.

6. Spinach and Avocado Salad with Citrus Dressing:

Combine baby spinach, sliced avocados, red onion slices, and orange segments in a bowl. Dress with a kidney-friendly citrus dressing made from orange juice, lemon juice, olive oil, and a hint of honey or agave syrup.

7. Asian-Inspired Cabbage Salad with Ginger-Sesame Dressing:

Shred cabbage, carrots, and snow peas, and toss them together in a bowl.

Drizzle with a kidney-friendly ginger-sesame dressing made from sesame oil, rice vinegar, ginger, garlic, and a touch of low-sodium soy sauce.

8. Protein-Packed Lentil Salad with Mustard Dressing:
Mix cooked lentils with diced cucumbers, cherry tomatoes, red bell peppers, and chopped parsley.
Toss with a kidney-friendly mustard dressing made from Dijon mustard, apple cider vinegar, olive oil, and a hint of maple syrup.

These vibrant salads paired with kidney-friendly dressings offer a symphony of flavors while ensuring a mindful approach to kidney health. Adjust ingredients as needed based on individual dietary requirements and preferences.

Hearty Lunch Wraps and Sandwiches

Hearty lunch wraps and sandwiches present a canvas for a delightful blend of flavors, textures, and nutrients while catering to a kidney-friendly diet. Here are some delectable ideas for wraps and sandwiches:

1. Grilled Chicken Caesar Wrap:

Fill a whole-grain wrap with grilled chicken breast, romaine lettuce, cherry tomatoes, and a kidney-friendly Caesar dressing made with yogurt or low-phosphorus mayo.

2. Turkey and Avocado Wrap:

Wrap sliced turkey breast, avocado slices, mixed greens, and a drizzle of kidney-friendly ranch dressing in a whole-grain wrap for a satisfying lunch option.

3. Veggie Hummus Wrap:

Spread hummus on a wrap and fill it with roasted vegetables like bell peppers, zucchini, and eggplant.
Add mixed greens and a sprinkle of feta cheese for extra flavor.

4. Tuna Salad Sandwich:

Prepare a kidney-friendly tuna salad with low-sodium tuna, diced celery, red onions, and a yogurt-based dressing.
Serve it on whole-grain bread with lettuce and tomato slices.

5. Caprese Panini:

Layer sliced tomatoes, fresh mozzarella, and basil leaves on whole-grain bread.
Grill it until the cheese melts, and drizzle with a kidney-friendly balsamic reduction.

6. Black Bean and Quinoa Wrap:

Combine cooked quinoa with black beans, diced bell peppers, corn, and cilantro.

Wrap it in a whole-grain tortilla with a kidney-friendly salsa or guacamole.

7. Eggplant and Pesto Sandwich:

Roast eggplant slices and layer them on whole-grain bread with basil pesto, sliced tomatoes, and arugula for a flavorful vegetarian option.

8. Roast Beef and Horseradish Wrap:

Wrap thinly sliced roast beef with shredded lettuce, sliced red onions, and a kidney-friendly horseradish sauce in a whole-grain tortilla.

9. Mediterranean Veggie Sandwich:

Spread hummus on whole-grain bread and top it with sliced cucumbers, roasted red peppers, Kalamata olives, and feta cheese for a flavorful option.

10. Chicken Salad Wrap:

Make a kidney-friendly chicken salad with diced chicken, grapes, celery, and a yogurt-based dressing.
Wrap it in a whole-grain tortilla with lettuce leaves.

These hearty lunch wraps and sandwiches offer a delightful mix of ingredients, ensuring both taste and kidney-friendly choices. Adjust the fillings and condiments based on personal preferences and dietary requirements for a satisfying meal.

Creative Lunchbox Ideas for Work or School

Here's a spectrum of creative and nutritious lunchbox ideas perfect for work or school, combining variety, flavor, and kidney-friendly choices:

1. DIY Salad Jar:

Layer kidney-friendly vegetables, such as cherry tomatoes, cucumbers, bell peppers, and mixed greens, in a mason jar.

Pack a separate container with kidney-friendly dressing to add just before eating to keep the salad fresh and crisp.

2. Pita Pocket with Hummus and Veggies:

Fill whole-grain pita pockets with kidney-friendly hummus, shredded carrots, sliced cucumbers, and baby spinach for a nutritious and portable meal.

3. Sushi Rolls with Quinoa:

Roll cooked quinoa, avocado slices, cucumber sticks, and cooked shrimp or imitation crab in nori sheets to create homemade sushi rolls.

Serve with low-sodium soy sauce or a kidney-friendly dipping sauce.

4. DIY Bento Box:

Create a bento box with compartments filled with kidney-friendly options like sliced fruits, cubed cheese, whole-grain crackers, mixed nuts, and carrot sticks for a balanced and varied meal.

5. Mason Jar Soup:

Prepare a kidney-friendly soup (such as vegetable or chicken noodle) and pour it into a thermos or mason jar.
Pack whole-grain crackers or a small side salad to accompany the soup.

6. Rainbow Veggie Wraps:

Spread low-sodium cream cheese or hummus on whole-grain wraps and fill them with a rainbow of kidney-friendly veggies—shredded carrots, bell peppers, spinach, and sliced tomatoes.

7. Protein-Packed Quinoa Salad:

Toss cooked quinoa with kidney-friendly ingredients like diced chicken, cherry

tomatoes, chopped cucumbers, and feta cheese.
Dress it with a kidney-friendly vinaigrette or lemon juice and olive oil.

8. Yogurt Parfait Jar:

Layer low-phosphorus yogurt with kidney-friendly fruits like berries, diced apples, and a sprinkle of granola or nuts in a portable jar for a quick and nutritious snack or light lunch.

9. Turkey and Cheese Roll-Ups:

Roll turkey slices around low-phosphorus cheese slices and include a side of whole-grain crackers or carrot sticks for a protein-rich and satisfying lunch option.

10. DIY Pasta Salad Cup:

Prepare a kidney-friendly pasta salad with whole-grain pasta, kidney-friendly vegetables, diced chicken or beans, and a kidney-friendly dressing.

Pack it in a reusable cup or container for a convenient and flavorful meal.

These creative lunchbox ideas offer a mix of nutrients, flavors, and textures, ensuring both nourishment and variety for a fulfilling meal at work or school while being mindful of kidney-friendly choices. Adjust ingredients based on personal preferences and dietary requirements for a satisfying lunch on-the-go.

7. Wholesome Dinners for CKD

Slow Cooker and Instant Pot Meals

Slow cooker and Instant Pot meals are convenient, time-saving, and versatile, offering a range of delicious options. Here's a selection of kidney-friendly recipes suitable for both appliances:

Slow Cooker Meals:

1. Slow Cooker Chicken Chili:

Combine diced chicken, kidney beans (rinsed to reduce potassium), low-sodium chicken broth, diced tomatoes, onions, bell peppers, and kidney-friendly spices in a slow cooker.

Cook on low for 6-8 hours for a hearty and flavorful chili.

2. Beef Stew:

Mix beef chunks with low-phosphorus vegetables like carrots, potatoes, onions, and celery in the slow cooker.

Add low-sodium beef broth, kidney-friendly herbs, and spices. Cook on low for 7-8 hours for a comforting stew.

3. Vegetarian Lentil Soup:

Combine lentils, low-phosphorus vegetables (like carrots, celery, and spinach), onions, garlic, and low-sodium vegetable broth in the slow cooker.

Cook on low for 6-8 hours for a nutritious and kidney-friendly soup.

4. Pulled Pork Tacos:

Place pork shoulder, low-sodium barbecue sauce, onions, and kidney-friendly seasonings in the slow cooker.

Cook on low for 8 hours, then shred the pork and serve in whole-grain tortillas with kidney-friendly toppings like shredded lettuce and diced tomatoes.

5. Slow Cooker Ratatouille:

Layer sliced eggplant, zucchini, bell peppers, onions, and tomatoes in the slow cooker.

Add kidney-friendly herbs, such as thyme and basil, and cook on low for 6 hours for a flavorful vegetable dish.

Instant Pot Meals:

1. Instant Pot Chicken and Vegetable Soup:
Combine diced chicken, low-phosphorus vegetables (like carrots, celery, and green beans), onions, garlic, low-sodium chicken broth, and kidney-friendly seasonings in the Instant Pot.
Cook on high pressure for 10 minutes for a quick and comforting soup.

2. Quinoa and Black Bean Stew:
Mix quinoa, black beans (rinsed), low-phosphorus vegetables (such as bell peppers, corn, and tomatoes), onions, garlic, low-sodium vegetable broth, and kidney-friendly spices in the Instant Pot.
Cook on high pressure for 8 minutes for a protein-packed stew.

3. Instant Pot Lemon Herb Chicken:

Marinate chicken breasts with lemon juice, herbs, garlic, and a touch of olive oil.

Cook on high pressure for 10 minutes for flavorful and tender chicken.

4. Instant Pot Vegetable Curry:

Combine kidney-friendly vegetables like cauliflower, potatoes, carrots, and peas with curry paste, coconut milk, onions, and garlic in the Instant Pot.

Cook on high pressure for 5 minutes for a fragrant and tasty curry.

5. Instant Pot Beef and Broccoli:

Mix beef strips, low-sodium soy sauce, garlic, ginger, broccoli florets, onions, and kidney-friendly seasonings in the Instant Pot.

Cook on high pressure for 10 minutes for a savory and nutritious dish.

These slow cooker and Instant Pot meal ideas offer a diverse range of kidney-friendly options that are both convenient and packed with flavor. Adjust ingredients to suit individual dietary needs and preferences for a delightful and nourishing meal.

Renal-Friendly Pasta and Rice Dishes

Here's a selection of renal-friendly pasta and rice dishes that are flavorful, nutritious, and mindful of kidney health:

Renal-Friendly Pasta Dishes:

1. Pasta Primavera:

Combine whole-grain pasta with kidney-friendly vegetables like bell peppers, broccoli, carrots, and cherry tomatoes.
Toss with a kidney-friendly garlic and olive oil sauce, flavored with herbs like basil and oregano.

2. Mushroom and Spinach Pasta:

Sauté mushrooms, spinach, and garlic in olive oil. Toss with cooked whole-grain pasta and kidney-friendly herbs like thyme or rosemary.

3. Lemon Garlic Shrimp Pasta:

Sauté shrimp in olive oil with garlic, lemon zest, and kidney-friendly spices.

Mix with cooked whole-grain pasta, fresh parsley, and a splash of low-sodium chicken or vegetable broth.

4. Pesto Pasta with Chicken or White Beans:

Toss whole-grain pasta with kidney-friendly pesto (made from basil, pine nuts, garlic, olive oil, and Parmesan) and diced chicken or white beans.

5. Tomato Basil Pasta:

Sauté fresh tomatoes, garlic, and kidney-friendly herbs like basil and oregano in olive oil.

Toss with cooked whole-grain pasta and garnish with fresh basil leaves.

Renal-Friendly Rice Dishes:

1. Vegetable Fried Rice:
Sauté kidney-friendly vegetables like peas, carrots, bell peppers, and onions in a little sesame oil.
Mix with cooked brown rice, low-sodium soy sauce, and a sprinkle of green onions for a flavorful dish.

2. Lemon Herb Rice with Chicken or Tofu:
Cook brown rice with lemon zest, kidney-friendly herbs, and low-sodium chicken or vegetable broth.
Serve with grilled chicken or tofu for a protein-rich meal.

3. Mushroom Risotto:
Sauté mushrooms, onions, and garlic in a pan. Add arborio rice and kidney-friendly broth gradually while stirring until creamy.
Finish with a sprinkle of Parmesan cheese (in moderation).

4. Coconut Curry Rice:
Cook brown rice with kidney-friendly vegetables like cauliflower, bell peppers, and spinach in coconut milk and curry spices for a fragrant and tasty dish.

5. Herbed Rice Pilaf:
Sauté onions and kidney-friendly vegetables in a pan. Add cooked brown rice and kidney-friendly herbs like thyme, sage, and rosemary.

These renal-friendly pasta and rice dishes offer a delicious variety while prioritizing kidney health. Adjust ingredients and seasoning based on individual dietary needs and taste preferences for a delightful and nourishing meal.

Sheet Pan Dinners and Grilling Recipes

sheet pan dinners and grilling recipes are fantastic for easy preparation and delicious meals. Here's a selection of renal-friendly options for both:

Sheet Pan Dinners:

1. Baked Lemon Herb Chicken with Vegetables:

Place seasoned chicken breasts on a sheet pan with kidney-friendly vegetables like carrots, bell peppers, and Brussels sprouts. Drizzle with olive oil, lemon juice, and herbs. Bake until chicken is cooked through and vegetables are tender.

2. Salmon and Asparagus Bake:

Arrange salmon fillets and asparagus spears on a sheet pan.
Drizzle with a kidney-friendly marinade of olive oil, garlic, lemon zest, and dill. Bake until the salmon is cooked and asparagus is tender.

3. Roasted Turkey Breast with Root Vegetables:

Season turkey breast and place it on a sheet pan surrounded by kidney-friendly root vegetables like carrots, parsnips, and sweet potatoes.

Drizzle with olive oil and herbs. Roast until the turkey is cooked and vegetables are caramelized.

4. Baked Tofu with Mixed Veggies:

Toss cubed tofu with kidney-friendly vegetables such as broccoli, cauliflower, and bell peppers on a sheet pan.

Season with a kidney-friendly marinade or spices. Bake until tofu is golden and veggies are tender.

5. Lemon Garlic Shrimp with Cherry Tomatoes and Zucchini:

Place shrimp, cherry tomatoes, and sliced zucchini on a sheet pan.

Drizzle with a kidney-friendly mixture of olive oil, lemon juice, garlic, and herbs.

Roast until the shrimp are pink and vegetables are tender.

Grilling Recipes:

1. Grilled Chicken Kebabs:
Skewer chunks of chicken breast, bell peppers, onions, and cherry tomatoes.
Brush with a kidney-friendly marinade of olive oil, lemon juice, garlic, and herbs. Grill until chicken is cooked and veggies are charred.

2. Grilled Vegetable Platter:
Grill kidney-friendly vegetables such as eggplant, zucchini, bell peppers, and mushrooms.
Drizzle with a kidney-friendly balsamic glaze or olive oil and herbs for a flavorful side dish.

3. Citrus-Marinated Tuna Steaks:

Marinate tuna steaks in a mixture of citrus juice (lemon, lime, or orange), olive oil, garlic, and herbs.

Grill until the tuna is cooked to your desired doneness.

4. Portobello Mushroom Burgers:

Marinate portobello mushroom caps in a kidney-friendly mixture of balsamic vinegar, olive oil, garlic, and herbs.

Grill until tender and serve on whole-grain buns with kidney-friendly toppings like lettuce, tomatoes, and avocado.

5. Grilled Veggie Skewers:

Skewer kidney-friendly vegetables like cherry tomatoes, onions, bell peppers, and mushrooms.

Brush with a kidney-friendly marinade and grill until the vegetables are lightly charred.

These sheet pan dinners and grilling recipes offer a diverse range of kidney-friendly options, making meal preparation both convenient and delicious. Adjust seasoning and ingredients based on individual dietary needs and preferences for a flavorful and satisfying meal.

8. Snacks, Sides, and Desserts

Nutritious Snacks with Low Potassium

Here are some nutritious snack ideas that are low in potassium:

1. Rice Cakes with Almond Butter: Spread a thin layer of almond butter on rice cakes for a satisfying and low-potassium snack.

2. Air-Popped Popcorn: Enjoy air-popped popcorn seasoned with herbs like garlic powder, paprika, or a sprinkle of Parmesan cheese for a low-potassium treat.

3. Carrot Sticks with Hummus: Dip carrot sticks into a portion-controlled amount of low-potassium hummus for a crunchy and nutritious snack.

4. Cottage Cheese with Apples: Pair a small serving of low-potassium cottage cheese with sliced apples for a balanced and tasty snack option.

5. Yogurt Bark: Mix plain, low-potassium yogurt with a small amount of honey and spread it on a baking sheet. Freeze and break into pieces for a refreshing snack.

6. Rice Crackers with Tuna: Top low-potassium rice crackers with a bit of canned tuna for a protein-rich and low-potassium snack.

7. Celery Sticks with Cream Cheese: Fill celery sticks with a light spread of low-potassium cream cheese for a satisfying and crunchy snack.

8. Roasted Chickpeas: Roast chickpeas seasoned with kidney-friendly spices like cumin or paprika for a crunchy and protein-packed snack.

9. Pretzels with Mustard: Enjoy a small serving of pretzels with a side of low-potassium mustard for a tangy and low-potassium snack.

10. Graham Crackers with Seed Butter: Spread a thin layer of seed butter (such as sunflower seed butter) on graham crackers for a delicious and low-potassium snack option.

These snack ideas provide variety while being mindful of potassium intake. Always consider portion sizes and individual dietary restrictions when incorporating snacks into a kidney-friendly diet.

Vegetable-Based Side Dishes

Here's a variety of vegetable-based side dishes that are flavorful and versatile while being kidney-friendly:

1. Roasted Garlic Parmesan Broccoli: Toss broccoli florets with olive oil, minced garlic, a sprinkle of Parmesan cheese, and roast in the oven until tender and slightly crispy.

2. Sautéed Green Beans with Almonds: Sauté fresh green beans with slivered almonds in a bit of olive oil until beans are tender-crisp. Finish with a squeeze of lemon juice for brightness.

3. Mushroom and Spinach Sauté: Sauté sliced mushrooms and spinach in olive oil with garlic until wilted. Season with herbs like thyme or rosemary for added flavor.

4. Zucchini Noodles (Zoodles) with Pesto: Create zucchini noodles using a spiralizer and toss them in a kidney-friendly pesto sauce made from basil, garlic, pine nuts, olive oil, and Parmesan cheese.

5. Cauliflower Mash: Steam cauliflower florets and blend until smooth. Season with a touch of butter (in moderation), garlic powder, and herbs for a creamy and low-carb alternative to mashed potatoes.

6. Grilled Eggplant Slices: Brush eggplant slices with olive oil and grill until tender. Sprinkle with kidney-friendly herbs like basil and oregano for a tasty side dish.

7. Stir-Fried Bok Choy: Stir-fry bok choy with a bit of garlic, ginger, and low-sodium soy sauce until wilted but still crunchy for a nutritious Asian-inspired side.

8. Brussels Sprouts with Bacon: Sauté halved Brussels sprouts with diced bacon until crispy and caramelized for a flavorful and savory side dish.

9. Steamed Carrots with Herbs: Steam carrot sticks until tender and toss them with kidney-friendly herbs like parsley, dill, or chives for a simple and nutritious side.

10. Tomato Cucumber Salad: Combine sliced tomatoes and cucumbers with a kidney-friendly dressing made from olive oil, vinegar, garlic, and a sprinkle of herbs like basil or parsley for a refreshing side dish.

These vegetable-based side dishes offer a variety of flavors and textures while being mindful of kidney-friendly ingredients. Adjust seasonings and ingredients based on personal preferences and dietary needs for a delightful accompaniment to any meal.

Indulgent Yet Kidney-Friendly Desserts

Indulgent desserts that are also kidney-friendly can be delicious and satisfying. Here are some ideas for treats that fit the bill:

1. Baked Apples with Cinnamon: Core apples, sprinkle them with cinnamon, a touch of nutmeg, and bake until soft. Serve with a dollop of low-potassium whipped cream or a sprinkle of chopped nuts.

2. Berry Sorbet: Blend kidney-friendly berries (like raspberries, strawberries, or blueberries) with a touch of honey and a splash of lemon juice. Freeze the mixture in an ice cream maker or a shallow dish, stirring occasionally for a refreshing sorbet.

3. Dark Chocolate-Dipped Fruit: Dip slices of kidney-friendly fruits (like bananas, strawberries, or dried apricots) in melted dark chocolate (moderately low in potassium). Let them cool on parchment paper for a delectable treat.

4. Rice Pudding: Make a kidney-friendly rice pudding using low-potassium rice, low-phosphorus milk, and sweetened with a touch of honey or a low-potassium sweetener. Flavor it with cinnamon or vanilla.

5. Lemon Bars with Almond Flour Crust: Prepare a crust using almond flour and butter (in moderation), top it with a kidney-friendly lemon custard made with eggs, lemon juice, and a low-potassium sweetener.

6. Frozen Banana "Ice Cream": Blend frozen bananas with a splash of low-potassium milk until creamy. Add a touch of vanilla or cocoa powder for flavor variation.

7. Chia Seed Pudding: Mix chia seeds with low-phosphorus milk or a non-dairy alternative and sweeten it with a low-potassium sweetener. Let it sit overnight in the fridge. Top with kidney-friendly fruits or a sprinkle of cinnamon.

8. Angel Food Cake with Berries: Enjoy a slice of angel food cake (low in potassium) with kidney-friendly berries and a dollop of low-potassium whipped cream or Greek yogurt.

9. Meringue Cookies: Make meringue cookies using egg whites and a low-potassium sweetener. Add a touch of vanilla or cocoa powder for flavor and bake until crisp.

10. Pumpkin Custard: Prepare a pumpkin custard using pureed pumpkin, low-phosphorus milk, eggs, and sweetened with a low-potassium sweetener. Season it with cinnamon and nutmeg for a delightful dessert.

These desserts offer a mix of flavors and textures while being mindful of kidney-friendly ingredients. Always consider portion sizes and individual dietary restrictions when enjoying these treats as part of a renal diet.

9. Beverages and Drinks

Hydration Boosting Infusions and Mocktails

Hydration-boosting infusions and mocktails can be refreshing and enjoyable while helping to increase fluid intake. Here are some ideas:

Hydration-Boosting Infusions:

1. Citrus Mint Infusion: Combine sliced oranges, lemons, and fresh mint leaves in a pitcher of water and let it infuse in the refrigerator. The citrus adds flavor, while mint provides a refreshing twist.

2. Cucumber and Basil Infusion: Slice cucumbers and add them to a pitcher of water along with fresh basil leaves. Let it sit for a few hours in the fridge for a subtle and hydrating drink.

3.   Berry-Infused   Water: Mix kidney-friendly berries like strawberries, blueberries, or raspberries in water and let it infuse for a couple of hours. The berries infuse the water with a mild fruity flavor.

4. Watermelon Rosemary Infusion: Blend watermelon chunks with a sprig of fresh rosemary and add it to a jug of water for a subtly sweet and aromatic drink.

5. Pineapple and Coconut Water Infusion: Mix chunks of pineapple with coconut water and let it sit in the fridge for a tropical and hydrating infusion.

Hydration-Boosting Mocktails:

1. Cucumber Cooler: Blend cucumbers with a bit of lime juice, mint leaves, and a splash of sparkling water for a refreshing mocktail.

2. Virgin Mojito: Muddle fresh mint leaves with lime juice and a low-potassium sweetener. Top it up with soda water for a zesty and refreshing drink.

3. Watermelon Limeade: Blend watermelon chunks with lime juice and a touch of honey or a low-potassium sweetener. Strain the mixture and serve it over ice for a revitalizing mocktail.

4. Berry Spritzer: Muddle kidney-friendly berries with a splash of lemon juice, add sparkling water, and serve over ice for a bubbly and fruity drink.

5. Herbal Iced Tea: Brew caffeine-free herbal teas like hibiscus or chamomile and let them chill. Sweeten with a low-potassium sweetener and garnish with a slice of lemon for a flavorful and hydrating option.

These hydration-boosting infusions and mocktails offer a variety of flavors and are a great way to increase fluid intake while enjoying refreshing and tasty drinks.

Smoothies and Shakes for Kidney Health

Smoothies and shakes can be excellent additions to a kidney-friendly diet, providing nourishment while allowing for creativity and taste variety. Here are some ideas:

1. Berry Blast Smoothie:

Blend kidney-friendly berries like strawberries, blueberries, and raspberries with low-phosphorus yogurt or a non-dairy alternative. Add a splash of low-potassium juice for sweetness.

2. Green Power Smoothie:

Blend spinach or kale with banana (in moderation), low-phosphorus almond milk, and a scoop of protein powder for a nutrient-packed green smoothie.

3. Tropical Delight Smoothie:

Blend kidney-friendly fruits like pineapple, mango, and banana (in moderation) with coconut water or low-phosphorus orange juice for a refreshing tropical flavor.

4. Creamy Avocado Shake:

Combine ripe avocado, low-phosphorus milk or a non-dairy alternative, a touch of vanilla extract, and a low-potassium sweetener for a creamy and nutritious shake.

5. Protein-Packed Peanut Butter Shake:

Blend peanut butter (in moderation) with low-phosphorus yogurt or a non-dairy alternative, a banana (in moderation), and a scoop of protein powder for a filling and tasty shake.

6. Citrus-Berry Fusion Smoothie:

Blend kidney-friendly citrus fruits like oranges, along with berries and a splash of low-potassium juice or water for a zesty and refreshing drink.

7. Oatmeal Breakfast Smoothie:

Blend cooked oatmeal (cooled), low-phosphorus milk or a non-dairy alternative, a banana (in moderation), and a sprinkle of cinnamon for a hearty and filling smoothie.

8. Carrot Cake Smoothie:

Blend carrots with a banana (in moderation), low-phosphorus milk or a non-dairy alternative, a touch of cinnamon and nutmeg for a flavorful, dessert-like shake.

9. Pomegranate Blueberry Smoothie:

Combine pomegranate seeds, blueberries, low-phosphorus yogurt or a non-dairy alternative, and a splash of low-potassium juice for a vibrant and antioxidant-rich smoothie.

10. Almond Cherry Shake:
Blend low-phosphorus almond milk with cherries, a touch of almond extract, and a low-potassium sweetener for a nutty and fruity shake.

These smoothies and shakes offer a range of flavors and nutrient profiles while being mindful of kidney-friendly ingredients.

Herbal Teas and Coffee Alternatives

Herbal teas and coffee alternatives offer flavorful options that can be enjoyed while maintaining a kidney-friendly diet. Here are some suggestions:

Herbal Teas:

1. Chamomile Tea: Known for its calming properties, chamomile tea is caffeine-free and offers a soothing and mild flavor.

2. Peppermint Tea: Refreshing and invigorating, peppermint tea is caffeine-free and aids in digestion.

3. Hibiscus Tea: Vibrant and tart, hibiscus tea is rich in antioxidants and has a pleasantly tangy taste.

4. Ginger Tea: Warming and spicy, ginger tea can aid in digestion and provide a soothing effect on the stomach.

5. Rooibos Tea: Naturally caffeine-free and slightly sweet, rooibos tea has a mild and earthy flavor.

6. Lemon Balm Tea: Delicately citrusy and calming, lemon balm tea is caffeine-free and promotes relaxation.

7. Dandelion Root Tea: Often used to support kidney health, dandelion root tea is caffeine-free and has a slightly nutty taste.

Coffee Alternatives:

1. Chicory Coffee: Made from roasted chicory root, it provides a rich and slightly bitter flavor reminiscent of coffee.

2. Herbal Coffee Blends: Various brands offer herbal coffee blends that mimic the taste of coffee without the caffeine, utilizing ingredients like roasted grains, nuts, and herbs.

3. Decaffeinated Coffee: While not entirely caffeine-free, decaffeinated coffee contains significantly less caffeine and can be an option for those seeking a milder effect.

4. Barley Coffee: Made from roasted barley grains, this alternative has a nutty and slightly bitter flavor, resembling the taste of coffee.

5. Carob-based Drinks: Carob-based beverages offer a mild and slightly sweet taste, often used as a caffeine-free alternative to cocoa or coffee.

These herbal teas and coffee alternatives provide a range of flavors and benefits without the caffeine content, making them suitable options for a kidney-friendly diet. Always consider individual tolerances and consult with a healthcare professional if you have specific dietary concerns or conditions.

10. Nutritional Therapy and Supplemental Support

Vitamins and Minerals in CKD Management

In chronic kidney disease (CKD), managing vitamins and minerals is crucial to maintain overall health. Here's an overview of key considerations:

1. Vitamin D: CKD often leads to decreased activation of vitamin D, impacting bone health. Supplementation with active vitamin D or vitamin D analogs may be necessary to maintain bone strength.

2. Calcium: As kidney function declines, the body's ability to regulate calcium diminishes. High levels of phosphorus in CKD can lead to calcium leaching from bones. Adjusting calcium intake through diet or supplements is essential to maintain balance.

3. Phosphorus: Elevated phosphorus levels in CKD can contribute to bone problems and cardiovascular complications. Monitoring phosphorus intake through diet (limiting high-phosphorus foods) and using phosphate binders can help manage levels.

4. Potassium: Impaired kidney function can cause potassium levels to rise, leading to heart and muscle issues. Regulating potassium intake by avoiding high-potassium foods like bananas, oranges, and potatoes is important.

5. Iron: CKD patients may develop anemia due to reduced erythropoietin production. Iron supplements or adjustments in diet (consuming iron-rich foods) can help manage anemia.

6. B Vitamins: CKD often affects B vitamin levels, particularly B6, B9 (folate), and B12. Supplementation or dietary modifications may be necessary to address deficiencies.

7. Sodium: Managing sodium intake is crucial in CKD to control blood pressure and fluid retention. Reducing salt intake and choosing low-sodium alternatives are beneficial.

Monitoring these vitamins and minerals is integral in CKD management. However, individual requirements can vary significantly, so personalized guidance from healthcare professionals or registered dietitians is essential for proper management and supplementation. Regular monitoring of blood levels and adjusting intake accordingly is key to supporting kidney health in CKD.

Herbal and Dietary Supplements

In chronic kidney disease (CKD), using herbal and dietary supplements should be approached cautiously, as they can interact with medications or exacerbate kidney issues. However, some supplements might have potential benefits when used under medical supervision:

1. Omega-3 Fatty Acids: Found in fish oil supplements, omega-3s may help reduce inflammation and cardiovascular risk in CKD patients.

2. Coenzyme Q10 (CoQ10): Known for its antioxidant properties, CoQ10 might benefit some individuals with CKD, particularly those on certain medications.

3. Red Clover: This herb might have antioxidant effects and could potentially assist in managing certain symptoms related to CKD.

4. Garlic: Some studies suggest that garlic supplements may aid in reducing blood pressure and inflammation, but use with caution, especially if taking anticoagulant medications.

5. Astragalus: Often used in traditional Chinese medicine, astragalus might have immune-boosting effects, but its safety and efficacy in CKD aren't well-established.

6. Probiotics: Supporting gut health may be beneficial for individuals with CKD. Probiotics could potentially help manage gastrointestinal issues and improve overall well-being.

7. Cranberry: Cranberry supplements might assist in preventing urinary tract infections (UTIs), which can be a concern in CKD.

It's crucial to emphasize that using supplements in CKD requires medical guidance. Some supplements might interfere with medications, exacerbate kidney issues, or cause side effects.

Additionally, dosage and purity of supplements can vary widely among brands, which could impact their effectiveness and safety.

Always consult healthcare professionals, including nephrologists or registered dietitians, before adding any herbal or dietary supplements to a CKD management plan. They can provide personalized advice based on individual health status, medications, and specific nutritional needs. Regular monitoring and assessments are vital to ensure safe and beneficial use of supplements in CKD.

Role of Nutritional Therapy in Treatment

Nutritional therapy plays a pivotal role in the treatment of chronic kidney disease (CKD), aiming to manage symptoms, slow disease progression, and maintain overall health. Here are key aspects of its role:

1. **Managing Nutrient Intake:**
Nutritional therapy focuses on regulating intake of nutrients like protein, sodium, phosphorus, potassium, and fluids. This helps prevent complications associated with imbalances in these elements.

2. **Slowing Disease Progression**:
Controlling protein intake, especially in advanced stages of CKD, can reduce the workload on the kidneys and slow disease progression.

3. **Blood Pressure and Fluid Management:** Dietary adjustments, particularly in sodium and fluid intake, help manage blood pressure and fluid retention, common issues in CKD.

4. **Managing Electrolyte Imbalances:**
Balancing potassium and phosphorus intake is crucial in preventing complications related to electrolyte imbalances, such as heart and bone issues.

5. Addressing Anemia: Nutritional therapy includes managing iron, B vitamins, and erythropoietin-stimulating agents to address anemia, common in CKD.

6. Supporting Bone Health: Calcium and vitamin D intake adjustments help support bone health, minimizing the risk of bone diseases associated with CKD.

7. Individualized Meal Planning: Tailoring meal plans to individual needs, taking into account stage of CKD, comorbidities, medications, and personal preferences, is vital for effective nutritional therapy.

8. Managing Symptoms and Quality of Life: Dietary modifications can alleviate symptoms like fatigue, nausea, and appetite loss, improving the overall quality of life for individuals with CKD.

Nutritional therapy in CKD is not a one-size-fits-all approach. It requires continuous monitoring, regular assessment, and adjustments based on individual needs and disease progression. Collaboration with a registered dietitian or nutritionist is essential to create personalized meal plans and provide ongoing support for managing CKD through diet and nutrition.

11. Lifestyle Modifications and Holistic Approaches

Physical Activity Recommendations

Physical activity is beneficial for individuals with chronic kidney disease (CKD) as it can improve overall health and quality of life. However, exercise recommendations may vary based on the individual's stage of CKD, overall health status, and any complications. Here are some general guidelines:

1. Consult Healthcare Professionals: Before starting any exercise regimen, individuals with CKD should consult their healthcare team, including nephrologists or primary care physicians, to ensure safety and appropriateness based on their condition.

2. Aim for Regular Exercise: Engaging in regular physical activity, within the limits of one's health, is beneficial. Aim for at least 150 minutes of moderate-intensity aerobic activity per week or as recommended by healthcare providers.

3. Variety in Exercise: Incorporate a mix of exercises, including aerobic activities (like walking, cycling, or swimming), strength training, and flexibility exercises. Avoiding high-impact activities might be advisable for those with advanced CKD or bone-related issues.

4. Listen to Your Body: Pay attention to how the body responds to exercise. If experiencing discomfort, fatigue, dizziness, or shortness of breath, it's essential to stop and rest.

5. Stay Hydrated: Proper hydration is crucial during exercise. Individuals with CKD need to be mindful of their fluid intake as excessive sweating or dehydration can impact kidney function.

6. Monitor Blood Pressure: Regularly monitor blood pressure before, during, and after exercise, especially for individuals with hypertension or cardiovascular issues associated with CKD.

7. Consider Personal Limitations: Depending on the stage of CKD, individuals may have limitations. Some may need to avoid heavy lifting or intense workouts due to the risk of injury or strain on the kidneys.

8. Individualized Approach: Exercise recommendations should be personalized. Healthcare professionals, including physical therapists or exercise physiologists, can help create a tailored exercise plan based on an individual's specific health status and limitations.

Regular physical activity, when done safely and in consultation with healthcare providers, can offer numerous benefits for individuals with CKD, including improved cardiovascular health, better muscle strength, increased energy levels, and enhanced overall well-being.

Stress Management Techniques

Managing stress is essential for overall well-being, especially for individuals dealing with chronic kidney disease (CKD). Here are some stress management techniques:

1. Mindfulness and Meditation: Practicing mindfulness or meditation can help reduce stress. Focus on the present moment, deep breathing, or try guided meditation sessions to relax the mind.

2. Physical Activity: Regular exercise, as recommended by healthcare providers, can release endorphins, improving mood and reducing stress levels. Choose activities suitable for your health condition.

3. Healthy Lifestyle: Eating a balanced diet, getting adequate sleep, and avoiding smoking and excessive alcohol consumption can contribute to stress reduction.

4. Relaxation Techniques: Explore relaxation methods such as deep breathing exercises, progressive muscle relaxation, or yoga to relax the body and mind.

5. Support Network: Seek support from friends, family, or support groups. Talking to others who understand what you're going through can be comforting.

6. Time Management: Organize tasks and prioritize responsibilities to manage stress related to time constraints. Break tasks into manageable steps to reduce feelings of overwhelm.

7. Hobbies and Activities: Engage in hobbies or activities you enjoy. Spending time on things you love can distract from stress and improve mood.

8. Counseling or Therapy: Consider seeking professional help if stress becomes overwhelming. Therapists or counselors can provide strategies to cope with stress effectively.

Managing stress in CKD requires a holistic approach that considers physical and emotional well-being. Implementing these techniques, alongside proper medical guidance, can significantly improve stress management and overall quality of life.

Integrative Approaches to Kidney Health

Integrative approaches to kidney health involve combining conventional medical treatments with complementary and alternative therapies to manage chronic kidney disease (CKD) and promote overall well-being. These approaches consider the whole person, including physical, mental, and emotional aspects. Here's a comprehensive overview:

1. Diet and Nutrition: A crucial aspect of integrative kidney health is a tailored diet. Working with a registered dietitian helps create a nutrition plan focusing on controlling protein, sodium, potassium, phosphorus, and fluid intake while ensuring adequate nutrition.

2. Herbal and Dietary Supplements: Some individuals incorporate herbs or supplements to complement conventional treatment. However, caution is necessary as some supplements can interact with medications or worsen kidney function. Always consult healthcare professionals before using any supplements.

3. Mind-Body Practices: Techniques like mindfulness meditation, yoga, tai chi, or deep breathing exercises can help manage stress, improve mental health, and potentially benefit kidney function indirectly by reducing stress-related complications.

4. Acupuncture and Acupressure: Some people explore acupuncture or acupressure to manage symptoms related to CKD, such as pain, nausea, or fatigue. Evidence on its direct impact on kidney function is limited, but these practices may offer symptomatic relief.

5. Exercise and Physical Therapy: Regular physical activity, tailored to an individual's health status, can improve overall well-being and cardiovascular health. Physical therapy may be beneficial for some individuals to address specific mobility or muscle-related issues.

6. Herbal Medicine and Traditional Practices: Traditional herbal medicine from various cultures might offer alternative approaches to support kidney health. However, their safety and efficacy in CKD management require thorough evaluation and medical supervision.

7. Stress Management and Emotional Support: Addressing stress through counseling, support groups, or relaxation techniques can positively impact mental health, which indirectly influences overall health, including kidney function.

8. Lifestyle Modifications: Integrative approaches emphasize lifestyle changes like smoking cessation, alcohol moderation, and adequate sleep, which can contribute to overall health and potentially benefit kidney function.

It's essential to approach integrative treatments for kidney health cautiously, ensuring they complement conventional medical care. Individual considerations, such as disease stage, comorbidities, and personal preferences, should guide the integration of these approaches into a comprehensive treatment plan. Collaborating with healthcare professionals, including nephrologists, dietitians, and integrative medicine practitioners, is vital for safe and effective integrative care.

12. Medications, Treatments, and Therapies

Pharmacological Interventions in CKD

Pharmacological interventions play a significant role in managing chronic kidney disease (CKD) by addressing complications, slowing disease progression, and managing symptoms. Here's a comprehensive overview:

1. Blood Pressure Management:

Angiotensin-Converting Enzyme (ACE) Inhibitors and Angiotensin II Receptor Blockers (ARBs): These medications help lower blood pressure and reduce proteinuria, protecting the kidneys from further damage.

Calcium Channel Blockers (CCBs) and Beta-Blockers: These medications may also be prescribed to control blood pressure in individuals with CKD.

2. Anemia Management:

Erythropoiesis-Stimulating Agents (ESAs): Recombinant forms of erythropoietin are prescribed to manage anemia in CKD by stimulating red blood cell production.

3. Phosphate Binders:

Calcium-Based or Calcium-Free Phosphate Binders: Prescribed to control phosphate levels in the blood, reducing the risk of bone and cardiovascular complications associated with high phosphate levels in CKD.

4. Vitamin D Analogs:

Active Vitamin D (Calcitriol) or Vitamin D Analogues: Used to manage bone health by regulating calcium and phosphorus levels in individuals with CKD who have low vitamin D.

5. Diuretics:

Loop Diuretics: Prescribed to manage fluid retention in individuals with CKD, particularly those with edema or fluid overload.

6. Statins:

Cholesterol-Lowering Medications (Statins): Used to manage dyslipidemia and reduce the risk of cardiovascular events in individuals with CKD.

7. Potassium Binders:

Sodium Polystyrene Sulfonate: Used to lower high potassium levels in individuals with CKD who are unable to control potassium through diet or other means.

8. Anticoagulants/Antiplatelet Medications:

Antiplatelet Agents or Anticoagulants: May be prescribed to reduce the risk of blood clots and related complications in certain high-risk CKD patients.

9. Pain Management:

Pain Medications: Prescribed cautiously to manage pain associated with kidney-related complications, with attention to potential kidney toxicity of certain pain relievers.

10. Immunomodulators:

Immunosuppressants: In specific cases, such as immune-mediated kidney diseases like lupus nephritis or certain types of glomerulonephritis, immunosuppressive drugs may be used to manage inflammation and preserve kidney function.

These pharmacological interventions aim to manage symptoms, slow disease progression, and reduce complications associated with CKD. However, medications should be prescribed and monitored by healthcare professionals considering individual health status, stage of CKD, comorbidities, and potential drug interactions or adverse effects. Regular monitoring and adjustments in treatment plans are crucial for optimal management of CKD.

Dialysis Modalities and Considerations

Dialysis is a vital treatment for individuals with end-stage kidney disease (ESKD) when their kidneys can no longer function adequately. There are two primary types of dialysis: hemodialysis (HD) and peritoneal dialysis (PD), each with different modalities and considerations.

1. Hemodialysis (HD):

Conventional In-Center Hemodialysis: Patients receive treatments at a dialysis center, usually three times a week, where blood is filtered through a machine called a dialyzer. This modality provides comprehensive care with medical staff oversight.

Home Hemodialysis: This method allows patients to perform dialysis at home, either daily or several times a week, under medical guidance. It provides flexibility in treatment schedules and greater independence.

Nocturnal Hemodialysis: Patients undergo longer and slower dialysis sessions overnight while sleeping, providing gentler treatment and more time for fluid and waste removal. It can improve quality of life and flexibility during the day.

Considerations for Hemodialysis:

Vascular Access: A crucial aspect is establishing a reliable access point, either through an arteriovenous fistula (AVF), arteriovenous graft (AVG), or central venous catheter (CVC), to allow blood flow to and from the dialysis machine.

Fluid and Dietary Restrictions: HD requires strict adherence to fluid and dietary restrictions to manage electrolyte levels and fluid balance between treatments.

Transportation and Schedule: Conventional in-center HD may require transportation to and from the dialysis center, impacting the patient's schedule.

2. Peritoneal Dialysis (PD):

Continuous Ambulatory Peritoneal Dialysis (CAPD): This method involves manual exchanges of dialysis fluid multiple times a day. Patients perform exchanges at home or work, providing flexibility in daily routines.

Automated Peritoneal Dialysis (APD): Patients use a machine called a cycler to perform automated exchanges overnight while sleeping. This modality offers more freedom during the day.

Considerations for Peritoneal Dialysis:

Catheter Placement: A catheter is surgically placed into the abdomen for the infusion and drainage of dialysis fluid. Proper care is crucial to prevent infections.

Dialysis Fluid Exchange: PD requires regular exchanges of dialysis fluid, necessitating good hygiene and following a strict schedule to maintain effectiveness.

Peritonitis Risk: PD carries a risk of peritonitis, an infection of the peritoneum. Proper training and strict adherence to aseptic techniques are essential to minimize this risk.

Potential Impact on Lifestyle: PD allows more flexibility but may require adjustments to work schedules and lifestyle due to the need for regular exchanges.

Choosing the appropriate dialysis modality depends on individual health, lifestyle, and preferences. Patient education, support from healthcare professionals, and consideration of various factors help determine the most suitable dialysis option for each individual. Regular monitoring and adherence to treatment plans are crucial for optimal outcomes in dialysis therapy.

Transplantation as a Treatment Option

Kidney transplantation is considered the optimal treatment for end-stage kidney disease (ESKD) as it offers the best chance for a better quality of life and long-term survival compared to dialysis. Here's a comprehensive overview of kidney transplantation:

1. Benefits of Kidney Transplantation:

Improved Quality of Life: Transplantation provides greater freedom and flexibility compared to regular dialysis treatments, allowing recipients to lead a more normal life.

Long-Term Survival: Successful kidney transplantation offers better long-term survival rates compared to remaining on dialysis.

Reduced Healthcare Costs: While the initial costs of transplantation are high, in the long run, it tends to be more cost-effective than lifelong dialysis treatments.

2. The Transplantation Process:

Evaluation: Patients undergo a thorough evaluation process to assess their suitability for transplantation. This involves medical tests, psychological assessments, and consultations to ensure they are fit for the procedure.

Waiting List: Patients deemed suitable are placed on a national waiting list for a deceased donor kidney. The wait time can vary significantly based on factors like blood type, tissue match, and availability of organs.

Living Donor Transplantation: Some patients have the option of receiving a kidney from a living donor, such as a family member, friend, or altruistic donor. This type of transplant offers several advantages, including shorter wait times and potentially better outcomes.

Transplant Surgery: The transplant surgery involves the surgical placement of the donated kidney into the recipient's body. It typically takes a few hours, and patients usually stay in the hospital for several days after the procedure.

3. Post-Transplant Care:

Immunosuppression: Recipients require lifelong medications to suppress the immune system and prevent rejection of the transplanted kidney. Regular monitoring of drug levels and adjustments are necessary to balance the risk of rejection and side effects.

Medical Surveillance: Recipients undergo regular check-ups, blood tests, and imaging studies to monitor kidney function, detect potential complications, and manage any issues promptly.

Lifestyle Adjustments: Patients are encouraged to adopt a healthy lifestyle, including a balanced diet, regular exercise, and avoiding smoking and excessive alcohol consumption to promote overall health and protect the transplanted kidney.

4. Potential Complications:

Rejection: The body's immune system may recognize the transplanted kidney as foreign and attempt to reject it. Immunosuppressive medications aim to prevent this, but rejection remains a potential complication.

Infections: Due to suppressed immunity, transplant recipients are at a higher risk of infections. Preventive measures and prompt treatment of infections are essential.

Side Effects of Medications: Immunosuppressive drugs can have side effects, including increased susceptibility to certain cancers, high blood pressure, diabetes, and bone thinning.

Kidney transplantation offers an excellent option for eligible candidates with ESKD, providing the opportunity for a better quality of life and long-term survival. However, it requires lifelong medical care, adherence to medications, and regular follow-ups to ensure the success and longevity of the transplanted kidney. Close collaboration with a transplant team and adherence to the recommended medical regimen are crucial for a successful outcome post-transplantation.

13. Coping Strategies and Support Systems

Coping with Lifestyle Changes

Coping with lifestyle changes, especially when managing a chronic condition like kidney disease, can be challenging. Here's a comprehensive guide on coping strategies:

1. Education and Understanding:

Knowledge is empowering. Learn about the condition, treatment options, and necessary lifestyle changes. Understanding the reasons behind lifestyle modifications can make them more manageable.

2. Acceptance and Adaptation:

Acknowledge the changes in life and accept them as a part of the new reality. Adaptation involves making gradual adjustments to accommodate these changes.

3. Support System:

Build a strong support network comprising family, friends, healthcare professionals, or support groups. Sharing experiences and receiving encouragement or advice can be immensely helpful.

4. Healthy Coping Mechanisms:

Explore stress-relieving activities like meditation, yoga, deep breathing, or mindfulness. Engaging in hobbies or activities that bring joy can act as healthy distractions.

5. Setting Realistic Goals:

Break down larger goals into smaller, manageable steps. Celebrate achievements, no matter how small, as they contribute to progress.

6. Communication:

Openly communicate with healthcare providers about concerns, challenges, or barriers faced in implementing lifestyle changes. They can offer guidance or modifications to the treatment plan.

7. Embracing a Positive Mindset:
Maintain a positive attitude and focus on what can be controlled rather than dwelling on what cannot. Seek inspiration from success stories or positive experiences of others.

8. Lifestyle Modifications:
Embrace lifestyle changes gradually. Focus on aspects like dietary adjustments, physical activity, managing stress, and adhering to treatment plans. Small changes over time can lead to significant improvements.

9. Seeking Professional Help:
Consider consulting a therapist, counselor, or psychologist if the lifestyle changes significantly impact mental health or if it becomes challenging to cope.

10. Time Management and Organization:

Effective time management and organization can help in incorporating new routines or tasks into daily life. Prioritize activities and set realistic schedules.

11. Patience and Self-Compassion:

Lifestyle changes take time to adapt to. Be patient with yourself and practice self-compassion. Acknowledge efforts made, even when progress seems slow.

12. Continuous Learning and Adjustment:

Stay open to learning and making adjustments along the way. Needs and circumstances change, requiring modifications in coping strategies and lifestyle adjustments.

Coping with lifestyle changes associated with managing kidney disease involves a multifaceted approach. It's essential to personalize coping strategies based on individual needs and preferences while seeking support from healthcare providers and loved ones. Gradual adaptation, persistence, and a positive mindset play crucial roles in successfully managing lifestyle changes.

Building a Support Network

Building a solid support network is crucial when navigating the challenges of kidney disease. Here's a comprehensive guide on establishing and nurturing a supportive circle:

1. Family and Friends:
Share your journey with loved ones. Their emotional support, understanding, and companionship can be incredibly comforting during difficult times.

2. Healthcare Team:

Develop a strong rapport with healthcare providers, including nephrologists, nurses, dietitians, and social workers. They offer medical guidance, support, and resources tailored to your needs.

3. Support Groups:

Join local or online support groups for kidney disease patients. Connecting with individuals who share similar experiences provides empathy, encouragement, and practical advice.

4. Patient Advocacy Organizations:

Engage with patient advocacy organizations focused on kidney health. These groups offer resources, educational materials, and advocacy opportunities to empower patients and their families.

5. Online Communities:

Participate in online forums, social media groups, or blogs dedicated to kidney disease. These platforms facilitate discussions, information sharing, and emotional support from a broader community.

6. Counselors or Therapists:

Consider counseling or therapy to address emotional challenges related to kidney disease. Professional guidance helps manage stress, anxiety, or depression that may arise from the diagnosis or treatment.

7. Religious or Spiritual Groups:

Seek support from religious or spiritual communities that offer comfort, guidance, and a sense of belonging. Many find solace and strength through faith-based connections.

8. Educational Workshops or Seminars:

Attend educational workshops or seminars focused on kidney health. These events provide valuable information, networking opportunities, and a chance to meet others facing similar situations.

9. Caregiver Support:

If you're a caregiver, seek support from caregiver-specific groups or resources. Taking care of yourself ensures you can better support your loved one with kidney disease.

10. Volunteering or Peer Support:

Engage in volunteering or offering peer support to others facing kidney disease challenges. Being a source of support for others can also reinforce your own coping strategies.

11. Community Resources:

Explore community centers, libraries, or local health organizations offering programs, workshops, or activities related to kidney health.

12. Personal Advocacy:

Advocate for yourself by actively engaging in your treatment plan, asking questions, and seeking clarification from healthcare professionals. Being proactive can empower you in managing your condition.

Establishing a diverse and robust support network provides various forms of assistance, encouragement, and understanding throughout your kidney disease journey.

Remember, nurturing these connections takes time, but they can be invaluable in enhancing your well-being and resilience in coping with the challenges of kidney disease.

Dealing with Emotional Challenges

Coping with emotional challenges that arise from kidney disease requires a multifaceted approach. Here's a comprehensive guide on dealing with these emotional hurdles:

1. Acknowledgment and Acceptance:

Accept and acknowledge your feelings. It's normal to experience a range of emotions such as sadness, frustration, fear, or anger. Recognizing these emotions is the first step towards managing them.

2. Education and Understanding:

Educate yourself about kidney disease. Understanding the condition, treatment options, and possible outcomes can alleviate anxiety and empower you to take proactive steps.

3. Support Network:

Build a strong support network. Lean on family, friends, support groups, or mental health professionals for emotional support, guidance, and a listening ear.

4. Open Communication:
Talk openly about your feelings with trusted individuals. Expressing your emotions can alleviate stress and help others understand what you're going through.

5. Professional Help:
Consider therapy or counseling. A therapist or psychologist can provide coping strategies, emotional support, and tools to manage stress, anxiety, or depression related to kidney disease.

6. Stress Management Techniques:
Practice relaxation techniques such as deep breathing exercises, meditation, mindfulness, or yoga. These practices help reduce stress and promote emotional well-being.

7. Healthy Lifestyle Habits:

Adopt healthy lifestyle habits. Eating a balanced diet, regular exercise, adequate sleep, and avoiding unhealthy coping mechanisms like excessive alcohol or tobacco can positively impact emotions.

8. Express Creativity or Hobbies:

Engage in activities or hobbies you enjoy. Creative outlets like art, music, writing, or gardening can serve as therapeutic tools to channel emotions.

9. Accepting Limitations and Setting Realistic Goals:

Accept the limitations imposed by kidney disease and set achievable goals. Focus on what you can control and celebrate small achievements.

10. Positive Self-Talk and Mindset:

Practice positive self-talk and maintain a hopeful outlook. Replace negative thoughts with positive affirmations to cultivate resilience.

11. Seeking Distraction and Enjoyment:

Distract yourself with activities you enjoy. Watching movies, reading, spending time in nature, or spending quality time with loved ones can provide relief from emotional distress.

12. Gratitude and Perspective:

Practice gratitude. Focus on what you're grateful for in life. Maintaining perspective can help navigate through difficult times.

Dealing with emotional challenges related to kidney disease involves a combination of self-awareness, seeking support, adopting healthy coping mechanisms, and being patient with yourself. Remember that managing emotions is an ongoing process, and it's okay to seek help when needed. Prioritizing emotional well-being is essential for overall health while navigating the complexities of kidney disease.

Conclusion

Empowering oneself through diet is a powerful strategy in managing and promoting better kidney health. It's evident that a well-planned, nutrient-balanced diet plays a pivotal role in supporting kidney function and mitigating complications associated with kidney disease. By understanding the impact of various nutrients, adhering to dietary guidelines, and making informed food choices, individuals can significantly enhance their well-being.

Taking charge of one's diet involves more than just following a set of restrictions; it's about embracing a lifestyle that prioritizes wholesome nutrition while navigating dietary limitations. Through collaboration with healthcare professionals, particularly registered dietitians specializing in kidney health, individuals can tailor their dietary plans to suit their specific needs, disease stage, and lifestyle preferences. This personalized approach fosters a sense of empowerment and enables individuals to make informed decisions regarding food choices, portion sizes, and meal planning.

Moreover, it's crucial to acknowledge the psychological aspect of dietary changes. Adapting to new eating habits can pose challenges, and the journey may be filled with emotional hurdles. However, by seeking support from a strong network, staying educated, addressing emotional barriers, and employing various coping strategies, individuals can navigate these challenges more effectively.

Ultimately, empowering oneself through diet for better kidney health is a continuous process that requires commitment, perseverance, and patience. It's about embracing the role of an active participant in one's health journey, understanding that each nutritious meal, each mindful choice, and each step toward a healthier lifestyle contributes to improved kidney function and overall well-being. By embracing this empowerment, individuals can take charge of their health, optimize kidney function, and pave the way for a more fulfilling life.